Easy Keto

Chaffle

Cookbook For Beginners

The Ultimate Guide On A Keto Chaffle Recipes To Burn Fat And Boost Metabolism.

Carol Gervais

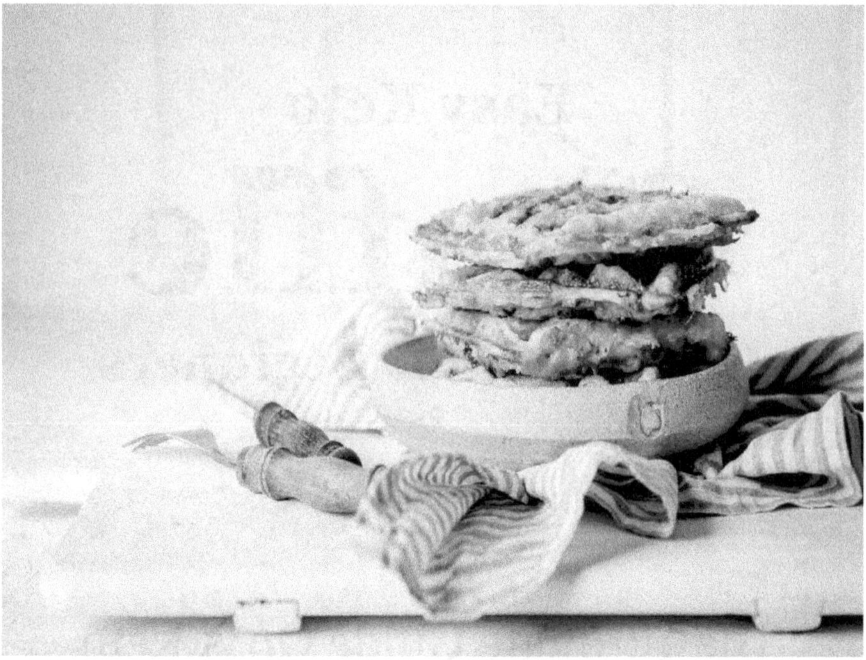

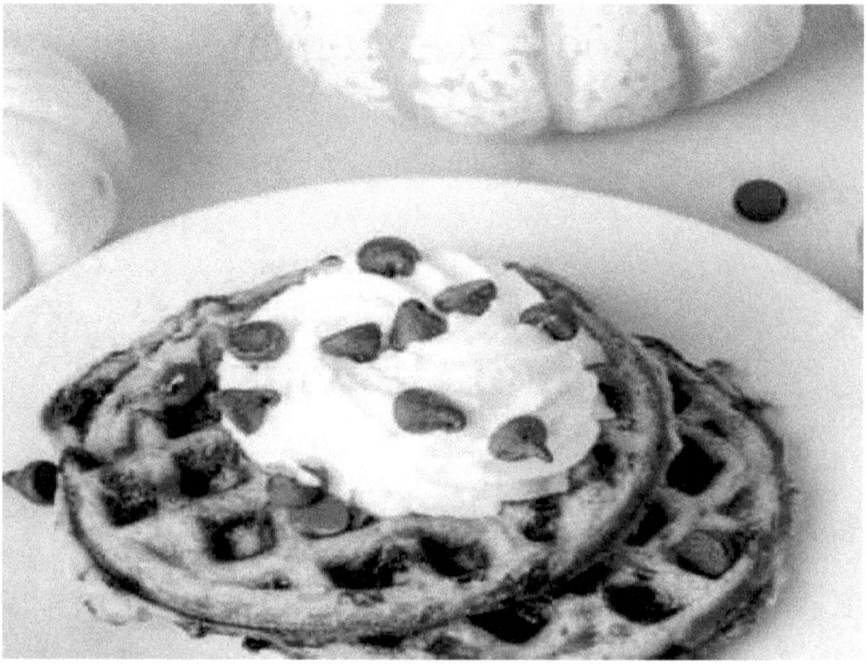

TABLE OF CONTENTS

TABLE OF CONTENTS.. 3

© COPYRIGHT 5

INTRODUCTION 7

KETOGENIC DIET AND ITS BENEFITS............................ 11

What is Ketogenic Diet?..11

Benefits of the Ketogenic Diet...11

Foods Allowed 14

Foods That Are Not Allowed 15

Volume (liquid) 17

Weight (mass)..18

Volume Equivalents (liquid)* 18

BREAKFAST CHAFFLE RECIPES....................................... 19

1.   Garlic and Parsley Chaffle 19

2.   Scrambled Eggs on A Spring Onion Chaffle 21

3.   Egg on A Cheddar Cheese Chaffle.......................23

4.   Avocado Chaffles Toast 25

5.   Cajun & Feta Chaffle 27

6.   Crispy Chaffles Plus Sausage 29

7.   Chili Chaffles 31

8.   Simple & Savory Chaffle 33

BASIC SANDWICH AND CAKE CHAFFLE RECIPES 35

9.   Strawberry Cream Sandwich Chaffles 35

10. Ham Sandwich Chaffle 37

11. Salmon and Cheese Sandwich Chaffles 39

12. Strawberry Cream Cheese Sandwich Chaffles ...41

13. Egg & Bacon Sandwich Chaffles............................43

14. Blueberry Peanut Butter Sandwich Chaffles.......45

15. Chocolate Sandwich Chaffles 47

16. Berry Sauce and Sandwich Chaffles.....................49

SWEET CHAFFLE RECIPES.. 51

17. Chocolate Cream Cheese Chaffles 51

18. Colby Jack Chaffles..53

19. Chaffle Birthday Cake..55

20. Chaffle-Churros..57

21. Strawberry Chaffle 59

22. Glazed Chaffles 61

23. Banana Nut Muffin 63

SAVORY CHAFFLE RECIPES.. 65

24. Hot Ham & Cheese Chaffles 65
25. Big Mac Chaffle 67
26. Japanese Style Chaffle Pizza 69
27. Keto Pepperoni Chaffle Pizza 71
28. Keto Cauliflower Onion Pizza Chaffle 73
29. BBQ Chicken Pizza Chaffle 75
30. Simple Vegetable Pizza Chaffle 77
31. Simple Savory Chaffles 79
32. Hot Pork Chaffles 81

MORE KETO CHAFFLE RECIPES 83

33. Crispy Bacon Chaffle 83
34. Almonds Crispy Chaffle 85
35. Olives Layered Chaffle 87
36. Cin-Cheese Chaffles with the Sauce 89
37. Fried Pickle Chaffle 91
38. Plain BBQ Crispy Chaffle 93
39. Bagel Chaffles 95
40. Celery and Cottage Cheese Chaffles 97

CONCLUSION 101

The following Book is reproduced below with the goal of providing information that is as accurate and reliable as possible. Regardless, purchasing this Book can be seen as consent to the fact that both the publisher and the author of this book are in no way experts on the topics discussed within and that any recommendations or suggestions that are made herein are for entertainment purposes only. Professionals should be consulted as needed prior to undertaking any of the action endorsed herein.

This declaration is deemed fair and valid by both the American Bar Association and the Committee of Publishers Association and is legally binding throughout the United States.

Furthermore, the transmission, duplication, or reproduction of any of the following work including specific information will be considered an illegal act irrespective of if it is done electronically or in print. This extends to creating a secondary or tertiary copy of the work or a recorded copy and is only

The information in the following pages is broadly considered a truthful and accurate account of facts and as such, any inattention, use, or misuse of the information in question by the reader will render any resulting actions solely under their purview. There are no scenarios in which the publisher or the original author of this work can be in any fashion deemed liable for any hardship or damages that may befall them after undertaking information described herein.

Additionally, the information in the following pages is intended only for informational purposes and should thus be thought of as universal. As befitting its nature, it is presented without assurance regarding its prolonged validity or interim quality. Trademarks that are mentioned are done without written consent and can in no way be considered an endorsement from the trademark holder.

INTRODUCTION

Keto Diet is a high-fat, low-carb diet that is an increasingly popular way to lose weight. Keto is short for "ketosis", which occurs when the body has depleted its sugar stores, so it burns stored fat instead of glucose in order to produce energy.

Losing weight on a keto diet sounds pretty easy; just eat a few bacon sandwiches and you'll be slimmer in no time. However, there are drawbacks to this diet, including very low levels of vegetables and fruit (so important for fiber and other nutrients) as well as constipation from lack of dietary fiber. Here are some tips:

- It's important to drink plenty of water, not only because you may be eating more sodium than you need, but because staying hydrated will help your body process proteins and fats more efficiently.

- For best results, stay away from most fruits and vegetables. Some berries are allowed; others aren't. Vegetables that are considered "low in carbs" or "leafy greens" are fine—but there is a difference between low-carb and high-fiber. As a rule of thumb, if it looks like it has the texture of tree bark or is covered with seeds or bulbs (e.g., artichokes), it probably has a lot of carbs and should be avoided.

- Be careful with spices, which tend to have a lot of sugar; salt is OK. It can be easy to go overboard on spices.

- Eat plenty of salmon, tuna and egg whites. Meat—including beef, chicken, pork and lamb—should comprise 20 to 25 percent of your total diet. (Be aware that "lean" meat is often not very lean. Be prepared to trim off most of that fat before cooking.) A little bacon or sausage is fine, too.

- Avoid condiments and sauces, including barbecue sauce and ketchup. These are full of sugar and other unhealthy ingredients.

- Drink mostly water (or unsweetened drinks such as tea or coffee). Try to avoid drinks with a lot of added sugar, like fruit juice or alcohol. If you choose to drink wine, go for the dry stuff—red wine is best.

Now, for Chaffles.

What is Chaffle?

Keto chaffle recipe is a versatile and easy-to-make low carb pancake that only requires 2 ingredients. It's a way to satisfy your sweet cravings while staying keto!

Chaffle is made from cheese and eggs. You will need grated cheddar cheese (use any kind of cheese you have on hand) and eggs, beaten together, then fried in a pan with butter or coconut oil.

Chaffles are perfect for a low carb breakfast, lunch or dinner and can be a treat right out of the pan, with butter!

Why Keto and Chaffle is a perfect combination?

Keto Chaffle is a great way to satisfy your sweet cravings while staying 100% in ketosis. It helps you feel fuller for longer but at the same time it's not a high carb treat.

Chaffle gives you a lot of energy and it's an easy way to prepare breakfast if you want it to be ready quickly when you get up or even if you're in a hurry so it can be prepared on the go without any issues.

Keto Chaffle tastes amazing plain, with butter or with any toppings you like and it can also be used as sandwich bread substitute.

KETOGENIC DIET AND ITS BENEFITS

What is Ketogenic Diet?

The ketogenic diet is a low-carb, high-fat diet. This means that the macronutrient ratio of your diet should consist mainly of fat and protein with only a small percentage of carbohydrates.

The idea behind the ketogenic diet is to force your body to use fat rather than glucose as its primary fuel source. When we are in ketosis, we can function on almost any fuel source.

Benefits of the Ketogenic Diet

The benefits of the ketogenic diet are as follows:

1. No need to count calories.

On this diet, you can eat as much as you want. Since there are no grains, the carbohydrates in the diet are very low, and so you will not take in many calories.

2. There is no need to spend a lot of money on expensive foods.

Since this diet is high in fat, one of the cheapest sources of fat is chicken thighs and legs and other skinless poultry parts or meats from around the animal, such as organ meats (heart, liver, etc.).

3. Low levels of Beta-hydroxybutyrate (ketone body) is suitable for brain health

The ketogenic diet can increase the level of ketone bodies by 10 times than normal dietary levels through fat metabolism.

4. Decreased risk of heart disease

Many people can lower their LDL (bad) cholesterol by 75-90% and triglyceride levels by 60%.

5. Less inflammation

Because there are no carbohydrates in the ketogenic diet, your body becomes very efficient at burning ketones as fuel. This is excellent news if you have an autoimmune disorder like rheumatoid arthritis or Crohn's disease because inflammation is often linked to autoimmune problems.

6. Fast weight loss

People usually start losing weight within two weeks of starting the diet.

7. Increased energy levels

The ketogenic diet can increase your energy levels because you will be consuming a high-fat diet with very few carbohydrates.

8. No constant hunger

When people are on a ketogenic diet, they are in "ketosis." This means that their bodies are using fat as an almost complete fuel source. This is the opposite of how most people function in a non-ketogenic state, which usually involves using carbohydrates (sugars) as a practically whole fuel source. Because the ketogenic diet is so different, the body is forced to use fat as its primary fuel source to function. This means you won't be hungry all the time once you get the hang of it.

9. No need for cheat meals

Since carbohydrates are reduced in this diet, cheating on the ketogenic diet will not help you lose weight because your body does not have carbohydrates stored to keep your metabolism running, being that fat is used instead of sugar/carbs.

10. No need to buy expensive supplements

Since the diet is not very restrictive, you won't need to buy many supplements besides vitamin D3 if you are deficient.

11. You can gain muscle and lose fat at the same time

When you do strength training with a ketogenic diet, the weight loss is due to body fat (adipose tissue), not muscle mass. Many people find it difficult to lose weight because they are losing muscle mass and body fat, which is not suitable for overall health. However, because this diet encourages protein consumption at every meal, as well as healthy fats, your amino acid intake will be sufficient to preserve your muscles without inhibiting your weight loss.

Foods Allowed

Here is the list of foods you can eat during the ketogenic diet:

1. Meat, poultry, fish, shellfish, and eggs from pasture-fed animals (animals are fed a grass-fed diet)
2. Fish and seafood caught in the wild
3. Eggs from pastured hens
4. Vegetables, including root vegetables such as beets and carrots and leafy greens such as spinach and kale.

5. Healthy fats such as coconut oil or olive oil that can be used in place of butter or other oils (11 grams per day maximum)

6. Nuts and seeds such as macadamia nuts, walnuts, and pumpkin seeds

7. Low to moderate amounts of dairy products such as yogurt and cheese

8. Non-starchy vegetables such as broccoli, cauliflower, and other cruciferous vegetables

9. Fruits

Foods That Are Not Allowed

Foods that are not allowed

When following the keto diet, you will want to avoid eating the following foods:

1. Grains including wheat, oats, rice, and corn

2. Sugar, including honey, maple syrup, and sugar in all its forms

3. Vegetable oils such as canola, sunflower, and soybean oil

4. Trans fats such as margarine and vegetable shortening

5. Juices and sugary drinks such as soda, fruit juices with added sugar or artificial sweeteners, or milk alternatives made with grains such as almond milk

6. Grain-based dairy products such as butter and yogurt

7. Legumes such as beans, soybeans, and peanuts

8. Starchy vegetables such as potatoes, peas, and corn

9. Processed foods of any kind, including sauces and any food that contains a high percentage of preservatives

10. Beer (pure alcohol)

11. Low-fat or nonfat dairy products such as yogurt and cheese (dairy products that are low in fat but have carbohydrates)

12. Fruit juices with added sugars or artificial sweeteners

Volume (liquid)

US Customary	Metric
1/8 teaspoon	.6 ml
1/4 teaspoon	1.2 ml
1/2 teaspoon	2.5 ml
3/4 teaspoon	3.7 ml
1 teaspoon	5 ml
1 tablespoon	15 ml
2 tablespoon or 1 fluid ounce	30 ml
1/4 cup or 2 fluid ounces	59 ml
1/3 cup	79 ml
1/2 cup	118 ml
2/3 cup	158 ml
3/4 cup	177 ml
1 cup or 8 fluid ounces	237 ml
2 cups or 1 pint	473 ml
4 cups or 1 quart	946 ml
8 cups or 1/2 gallon	1.9 liters
1 gallon	3.8 liters

Weight (mass)

US contemporary (ounces)	Metric (grams)
1/2 ounce	14 grams
1 ounce	28 grams
3 ounces	85 grams
3.53 ounces	100 grams
4 ounces	113 grams
8 ounces	227 grams
12 ounces	340 grams
16 ounces or 1 pound	454 grams

Volume Equivalents (liquid)*

3 teaspoons	1 tablespoon	0.5 fluid ounce
2 tablespoons	1/8 cup	1 fluid ounce
4 tablespoons	1/4 cup	2 fluid ounces
5 1/3 tablespoons	1/3 cup	2.7 fluid ounces
8 tablespoons	1/2 cup	4 fluid ounces
12 tablespoons	3/4 cup	6 fluid ounces
16 tablespoons	1 cup	8 fluid ounces
2 cups	1 pint	16 fluid ounces

BREAKFAST CHAFFLE RECIPES

1. Garlic and Parsley Chaffle

Preparation Time: 10 minutes

Cooking Time: 5 Minutes

Servings: 1

Ingredients:

- 1 large egg
- 1/4 cup cheese mozzarella
- 1 tsp. coconut flour
- ¼ tsp. baking powder
- ½ tsp. garlic powder
- 1 tbsp. minutes parsley
- For Serving
- 1 Poach egg
- 4 oz. smoked salmon

Directions:

1. Switch on your Dash minutes waffle maker and let it preheat.
2. Grease waffle maker with cooking spray.
3. Mix together egg, mozzarella, coconut flour, baking powder, and garlic powder, parsley to a mixing bowl until combined well.
4. Pour batter in circle chaffle maker.
5. Close the lid.

6. Cook for about 2-3 minutes Utes or until the chaffles are cooked.
7. Serve with smoked salmon and poached egg.
8. Enjoy!

Nutrition:

- Protein: 45% 140 kcal
- Fat: 51% 160 kcal
- Carbohydrates: 4% 14 kcal

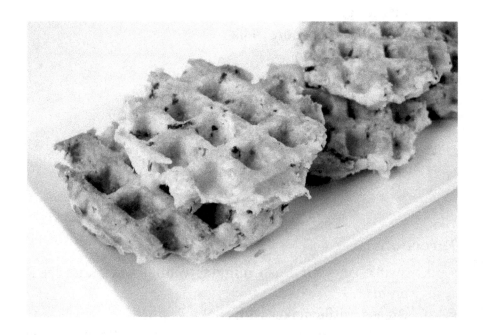

2. Scrambled Eggs on A Spring Onion Chaffle

Preparation Time: 10 minutes

Cooking Time: 7–9 Minutes

Servings: 4

Ingredients:

- Batter
- 4 eggs
- 2 cups grated mozzarella cheese
- 2 spring onions, finely chopped
- Salt and pepper to taste
- ½ teaspoon dried garlic powder
- 2 tablespoons almond flour
- 2 tablespoons coconut flour
- Other
- 2 tablespoons butter for brushing the waffle maker
- 6-8 eggs
- Salt and pepper
- 1 teaspoon Italian spice mix
- 1 tablespoon olive oil
- 1 tablespoon freshly chopped parsley

Directions:

1. Preheat the waffle maker.
2. Crack the eggs into a bowl and add the grated cheese.
3. Mix until just combined, then add the chopped spring onions and season with salt and pepper and dried garlic powder.
4. Stir in the almond flour and mix until everything is combined.

5. Brush the heated waffle maker with butter and add a few tablespoons of the batter.
6. Close the lid and cook for about 7–8 minutes depending on your waffle maker.
7. While the chaffles are cooking, prepare the scrambled eggs by whisking the eggs in a bowl until frothy, about 2 minutes. Season with salt and black pepper to taste and add the Italian spice mix. Whisk to blend in the spices.
8. Warm the oil in a non-stick pan over medium heat.
9. Pour the eggs in the pan and cook until eggs are set to your liking.
10. Serve each chaffle and top with some scrambled eggs. Top with freshly chopped parsley.

Nutrition:

- Calories: 194
- Fat: 14.7 g
- Carbs: 5 g
- Sugar: 0.6 g
- Protein: 1 g
- Sodium: 191 mg

3. Egg on A Cheddar Cheese Chaffle

Preparation Time: 10 minutes

Cooking Time: 7–9 Minutes

Servings: 4

Ingredients:

- Batter
- 4 eggs
- 2 cups shredded white cheddar cheese
- Salt and pepper to taste
- Other
- 2 tablespoons butter for brushing the waffle maker
- 4 large eggs
- 2 tablespoons olive oil

Directions:

1. Preheat the waffle maker.
2. Crack the eggs into a bowl and whisk them with a fork.
3. Stir in the grated cheddar cheese and season with salt and pepper.
4. Brush the heated waffle maker with butter and add a few tablespoons of the batter.
5. Close the lid and cook for about 7–8 minutes depending on your waffle maker.
6. While chaffles are cooking, cook the eggs.
7. Warm the oil in a large non-stick pan that has a lid over medium-low heat for 2-3 minutes
8. Crack an egg in a small ramekin and gently add it to the pan. Repeat the same way for the other 3 eggs.
9. Cover and let cook for 2 to 2 ½ minutes for set eggs but with runny yolks.
10. Remove from heat.

11. To serve, place a chaffle on each plate and top with an egg. Season with salt and black pepper to taste.

Nutrition:

- Calories: 4
- Fat: 34 g
- Carbs: 2 g
- Sugar: 0.6 g
- Protein: 26 g
- Sodium: 518 mg

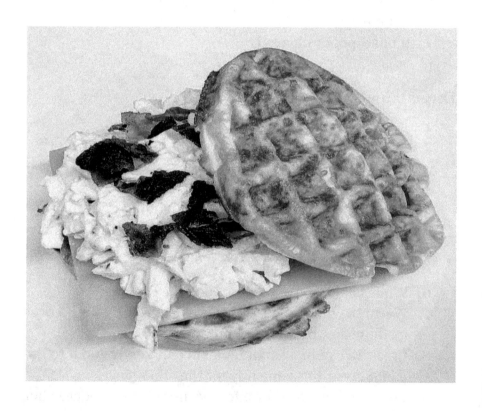

4. Avocado Chaffles Toast

Preparation Time: 10 minutes

Cooking Time: 10 Minutes

Servings:3

Ingredients:

- 4 tbsps. avocado mash
- 1/2 tsp lemon juice
- 1/8 tsp salt
- 1/8 tsp black pepper
- 2 eggs
- 1/2 cup shredded cheese
- For serving
- 3 eggs
- ½ avocado thinly sliced
- 1 tomato, sliced

Directions:

1. Mash avocado mash with lemon juice, salt, and black pepper in mixing bowl, until well combined.
2. In a small bowl beat egg and pour eggs in avocado mixture and mix well.
3. Switch on Waffle Maker to pre-heat.
4. Pour 1/8 of shredded cheese in a waffle maker and then pour ½ of egg and avocado mixture and then 1/8 shredded cheese.
5. Close the lid and cook chaffles for about 3 - 4 minutes Utes.
6. Repeat with the remaining mixture.
7. Meanwhile, fry eggs in a pan for about 1-2 minutes Utes.

8. For serving, arrange fried egg on chaffle toast with avocado slice and tomatoes.
9. Sprinkle salt and pepper on top and enjoy!

Nutrition:

- Protein: 26% 66 kcal
- Fat: 67% 169 kcal
- Carbohydrates: 6% 15 kcal

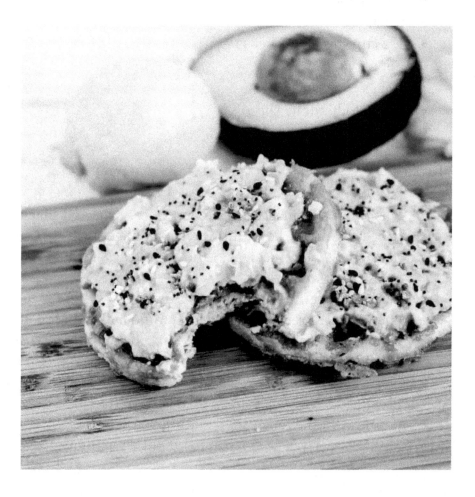

5. Cajun & Feta Chaffle

Preparation Time: 10 minutes

Cooking Time: 10 Minutes

Servings: 1

Ingredients:

- 1 egg white
- 1/4 cup shredded mozzarella cheese
- 2 tbsps. almond flour
- 1 tsp Cajun Seasoning
- FOR SERVING
- 1 egg
- 4 oz. feta cheese
- 1 tomato, sliced

Directions:

1. Whisk together egg, cheese, and seasoning in a bowl.
2. Switch on and grease waffle maker with cooking spray.
3. Pour batter in a preheated waffle maker.
4. Cook chaffles for about 2-3 minutes Utes until the chaffle is cooked through.
5. Meanwhile, fry the egg in a non-stick pan for about 1-2 minutes Utes.
6. For serving set fried egg on chaffles with feta cheese and tomatoes slice.

Nutrition:

- Protein: 28% 119 kcal
- Fat: 64% 2 kcal
- Carbohydrates: 7% 31 kcal

6. Crispy Chaffles Plus Sausage

Preparation Time: 10 minutes

Cooking Time: 10 Minutes

Servings: 2

Ingredients:

- 1/2 cup cheddar cheese
- 1/2 tsp. baking powder
- 1/4 cup egg whites
- 2 tsp. pumpkin spice
- 1 egg, whole
- 2 chicken sausage
- 2 slice bacon
- salt and pepper to taste
- 1 tsp. avocado oil

Directions:

1. Mix together all ingredients in a bowl.
2. Allow batter to sit while waffle iron warms.
3. Spray waffle iron with nonstick spray.
4. Pour batter in the waffle maker and cook according to the directions of the manufacturer.
5. Meanwhile, heat oil in a pan and fry the egg, according to your choice and transfer it to plate.
6. In the same pan, fry bacon slice and sausage on medium heat for about 2-3 minutes Utes until cooked.
7. Once chaffles are cooked thoroughly, remove them from the maker.
8. Serve with fried egg, bacon slice, sausages and enjoy!

Nutrition:

- Protein: 22% 86 kcal
- Fat: 74% 286 kcal
- Carbohydrates: 3% 12 kcal

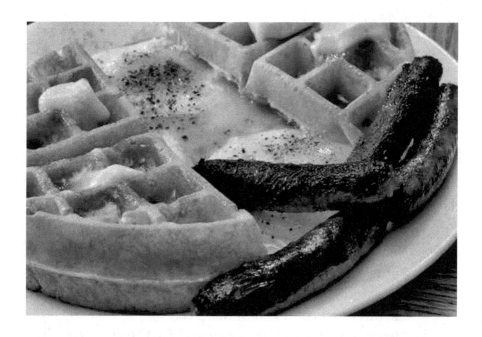

7. Chili Chaffles

Preparation Time: 10 minutes

Cooking Time: 7–9 Minutes

Servings: 4

Ingredients:

- Batter
- 4 eggs
- ½ cup grated parmesan cheese
- 1½ cups grated yellow cheddar cheese
- 1 hot red chili pepper
- Salt and pepper to taste
- ½ teaspoon dried garlic powder
- 1 teaspoon dried basil
- 2 tablespoons almond flour
- Other
- 2 tablespoons olive oil for brushing the waffle maker

Directions:

1. Preheat the waffle maker.
2. Crack the eggs into a bowl and add the grated parmesan and cheddar cheese.
3. Mix until just combined and add the chopped chili pepper. Season with salt and pepper, dried garlic powder and dried basil. Stir in the almond flour.
4. Mix until everything is combined.
5. Brush the heated waffle maker with olive oil and add a few tablespoons of the batter.
6. Close the lid and cook for about 7–8 minutes depending on your waffle maker.

Nutrition:

- Calories: 36
- Fat: 30.4 g
- Carbs: 3.1 g
- Sugar: 0.7 g
- Protein: 21.5 g
- Sodium: 469 mg

8. Simple & Savory Chaffle

Preparation Time: 10 minutes

Cooking Time: 7–9 Minutes

Servings: 4

Ingredients:

- Batter
- 4 eggs
- 1 cup grated mozzarella cheese
- 1 cup grated provolone cheese
- ½ cup almond flour
- 2 tablespoons coconut flour
- 2½ teaspoons baking powder
- Salt and pepper to taste
- Other
- 2 tablespoons butter to brush the waffle maker

Directions:

1. Preheat the waffle maker.
2. Add the grated mozzarella and provolone cheese to a bowl and mix.
3. Add the almond and coconut flour and baking powder and season with salt and pepper.
4. Mix with a wire whisk and crack in the eggs.
5. Stir everything together until batter forms.
6. Brush the heated waffle maker with butter and add a few tablespoons of the batter.
7. Close the lid and cook for about 8 minutes depending on your waffle maker.
8. Serve and enjoy.

Nutrition:

- Calories 352
- Fat: 27.2 g
- Carbs: 8.3 g
- Sugar: 0.5 g
- Protein: 15 g
- Sodium: 442 mg

BASIC SANDWICH AND CAKE CHAFFLE RECIPES

9. Strawberry Cream Sandwich Chaffles

Preparation Time: 6 minutes

Cooking Time: 6 Minutes

Servings: 2

Ingredients:

- Chaffles
- 1 large organic egg, beaten
- ½ cup mozzarella cheese, shredded finely
- Filling
- 4 teaspoons heavy cream
- 2 tablespoons powdered erythritol
- 1 teaspoon fresh lemon juice
- Pinch of fresh lemon zest, grated
- 2 fresh strawberries, hulled and sliced

Directions:

1. Preheat a mini waffle iron and then grease it.
2. For chaffles: in a small bowl, add the egg and mozzarella cheese and stir to combine.
3. Place half of the mixture into preheated waffle iron and cook for about 2–minutes.
4. Repeat with the remaining mixture.
5. Meanwhile, for filling: in a bowl, place all the ingredients except the strawberry slices and with a hand mixer, beat until well combined.

6. Serve each chaffle with cream mixture and strawberry slices.

Nutrition:

- Calories: 140
- Fat: 1.1g
- Carbs: 27.9g
- Protein: 4.7g
- Fiber: 10.9g

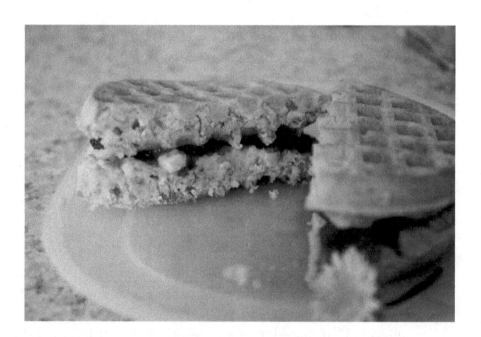

10. Ham Sandwich Chaffle

Preparation Time: 6 minutes

Cooking Time: 8 Minutes

Servings: 2

Ingredients:

- 1 organic egg, beaten
- ½ cup Monterrey Jack cheese, shredded
- 1 teaspoon coconut flour
- Pinch of garlic powder
- Filling
- 2 sugar-free ham slices
- 1 small tomato, sliced
- 2 lettuce leaves

Directions:

1. Preheat a mini waffle iron and then grease it.
2. For chaffles: In a medium bowl, put all ingredients and with a fork, mix until well combined. Place half of the mixture into preheated waffle iron and cook for about 3–4 minutes.
3. Repeat with the remaining mixture.
4. Serve each chaffle with filling ingredients.

Nutrition:

- Calories: 175
- Fat: 0.9g
- Carbs: 34.9g
- Protein: 6.7g
- Fiber: 7.5g

11.   Salmon and Cheese Sandwich Chaffles

Preparation Time: 6 minutes

Cooking Time: 24 Minutes

Servings: 4

Ingredients:

- Chaffles
- 2 organic eggs
- ½ ounce butter, melted
- 1 cup mozzarella cheese, shredded
- 2 tablespoons almond flour
- Pinch of salt
- Filling
- ½ cup smoked salmon
- 1/3 cup avocado, peeled, pitted, and sliced
- 2 tablespoons feta cheese, crumbled

Directions:

1. Preheat a mini waffle iron and then grease it.
2. For chaffles: In a medium bowl, put all ingredients and with a fork, mix until well combined. Place ¼ of the mixture into preheated waffle iron and cook for about 5–6 minutes.
3. Repeat with the remaining mixture.
4. Serve each chaffle with filling ingredients.

Nutrition:

- Calories: 352
- Fat: 10.0g
- Carbs: 51.5g
- Protein: 14.1g
- Fiber: 5.5g

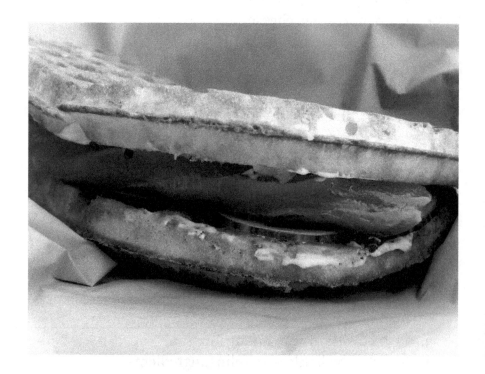

12. Strawberry Cream Cheese Sandwich Chaffles

Preparation Time: 6 minutes

Cooking Time: 10 Minutes

Servings: 2

Ingredients:

- Chaffles
- 1 organic egg, beaten
- 1 teaspoon organic vanilla extract
- 1 tablespoon almond flour
- 1 teaspoon organic baking powder
- Pinch of ground cinnamon
- 1 cup mozzarella cheese, shredded
- Filling
- 2 tablespoons cream cheese, softened
- 2 tablespoons erythritol
- ¼ teaspoon organic vanilla extract
- 2 fresh strawberries, hulled and chopped

Directions:

1. Preheat a mini waffle iron and then grease it.
2. For chaffles: in a bowl, add the egg and vanilla extract and mix well.
3. Add the flour, baking powder, and cinnamon, and mix until well combined.
4. Add the mozzarella cheese and stir to combine.
5. Place half of the mixture into preheated waffle iron and cook for about 4–minutes.
6. Repeat with the remaining mixture.

7. Meanwhile, for filling: in a bowl, place all the ingredients except the strawberry pieces and with a hand mixer, beat until well combined.
8. Serve each chaffle with cream cheese mixture and strawberry pieces.

Nutrition:

- Calories: 412
- Fat: 20.2g
- Carbs: 43.3g
- Protein: 21.6g
- Fiber: 13.1g

13. Egg & Bacon Sandwich Chaffles

Preparation Time: 6 minutes

Cooking Time: 20 Minutes

Servings: 4

Ingredients:

- Chaffles
- 2 large organic eggs, beaten
- 4 tablespoons almond flour
- 1 teaspoon organic baking powder
- 1 cup mozzarella cheese, shredded
- Filling
- 4 organic fried eggs
- 4 cooked bacon slices

Directions:

1. Preheat a mini waffle iron and then grease it.
2. In a medium bowl, put all ingredients and with a fork, mix until well combined. Place half of the mixture into preheated waffle iron and cook for about 3–5 minutes.
3. Repeat with the remaining mixture.
4. Repeat with the remaining mixture.
5. Serve each chaffle with filling ingredients.

Nutrition:

- Calories: 159
- Fat: 9.3g
- Carbs: 8.3g
- Protein: 10.4g
- Fiber: 1.6g

14. Blueberry Peanut Butter Sandwich Chaffles

Preparation Time: 6 minutes

Cooking Time: 10 Minutes

Servings: 2

Ingredients:

- 1 organic egg, beaten
- ½ cup cheddar cheese, shredded
- Filling
- 2 tablespoons erythritol
- 1 tablespoon butter, softened
- 1 tablespoon natural peanut butter
- 2 tablespoons cream cheese, softened
- ¼ teaspoon organic vanilla extract
- 2 teaspoons fresh blueberries

Directions:

1. Preheat a mini waffle iron and then grease it.
2. For chaffles: in a small bowl, add the egg and Cheddar cheese and stir to combine.
3. Place half of the mixture into preheated waffle iron and cook for about 5 minutes.
4. Repeat with the remaining mixture.
5. Meanwhile, for filling: In a medium bowl, put all ingredients and mix until well combined.
6. Serve each chaffle with peanut butter mixture.

Nutrition:

- Calories: 17
- Fat: 4g
- Protein: 9g

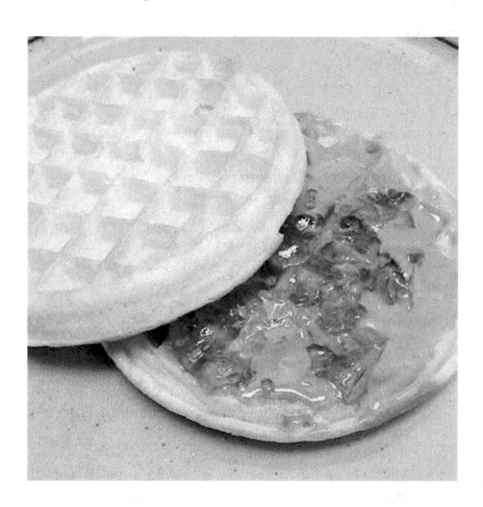

15. Chocolate Sandwich Chaffles

Preparation Time: 6 minutes

Cooking Time: 10 Minutes

Servings: 2

Ingredients:

- Chaffles
- 1 organic egg, beaten
- 1 ounce cream cheese, softened
- 2 tablespoons almond flour
- 1 tablespoon cacao powder
- 2 teaspoons erythritol
- 1 teaspoon organic vanilla extract
- Filling
- 2 tablespoons cream cheese, softened
- 2 tablespoons erythritol
- ½ tablespoon cacao powder
- ¼ teaspoon organic vanilla extract

Directions:

1. Preheat a mini waffle iron and then grease it.
2. For chaffles: In a medium bowl, put all ingredients and with a fork, mix until well combined. Place half of the mixture into preheated waffle iron and cook for about 3–5 minutes.
3. Repeat with the remaining mixture.
4. Meanwhile, for filling: In a medium bowl, put all ingredients and with a hand mixer, beat until well combined.
5. Serve each chaffle with chocolate mixture.

Nutrition:

- Calories: 102
- Fat: 22g
- Protein: 9g
- Sugar: 1g

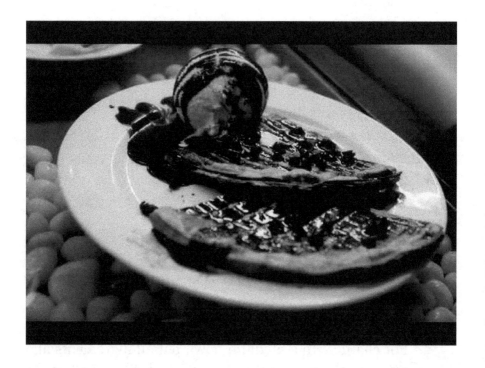

16.   Berry Sauce and Sandwich Chaffles

Preparation Time: 6 minutes

Cooking Time: 8 Minutes

Servings: 2

Ingredients:

- Filling
- 3 ounces frozen mixed berries, thawed with the juice
- 1 tablespoon erythritol
- 1 tablespoon water
- ¼ tablespoon fresh lemon juice
- 2 teaspoons cream
- Chaffles
- 1 large organic egg, beaten
- ½ cup cheddar cheese, shredded
- 2 tablespoons almond flour

Directions:

1. For berry sauce: in a pan, add the berries, erythritol, water and lemon juice over medium heat and cook for about 8– minutes, pressing with the spoon occasionally.
2. Remove the pan of sauce from heat and set aside to cool before serving.
3. Preheat a mini waffle iron and then grease it.
4. In a bowl, add the egg, cheddar cheese and almond flour and beat until well combined. Place half of the mixture into preheated waffle iron and cook for about 3–5 minutes.
5. Repeat with the remaining mixture.
6. Serve each chaffle with cream and berry sauce.

Nutrition:

- Calories: 548
- Fat: 20.7g
- Protein: 46g

SWEET CHAFFLE RECIPES

17. Chocolate Cream Cheese Chaffles

Preparation Time: 5 minutes

Cooking Time: 8 Minutes

Servings: 2

Ingredients:

- 1 large organic egg, beaten
- 1-ounce cream cheese, softened
- 1 tablespoon sugar-free chocolate syrup
- 1 tablespoon Erythritol
- ½ tablespoon cacao powder
- ¼ teaspoon organic baking powder
- ½ teaspoon organic vanilla extract

Directions:

1. Preheat a mini waffle iron and then grease it.
2. In a medium bowl, place all ingredients and with a fork, mix until well combined.
3. Place half of the mixture into preheated waffle iron and cook for about 4 minutes or until golden brown.
4. Repeat with the remaining mixture.
5. Serve warm.

Nutrition:

- Calories: 241 Kcal
- Total Fat: 2.1 g
- Saturated Fat: 0.7 g
- Carbohydrates: 43.3 g
- Fiber: 17.4 g
- Sugars: 16.5 g
- Protein: 11.3 g

18. Colby Jack Chaffles

Preparation Time: 8 minutes

Cooking Time: 6 Minutes

Servings: 1

Ingredients:

- 2 ounces Colby's jack cheese, sliced thinly in triangles
- 1 large organic egg, beaten

Directions:

1. Preheat a waffle iron and then grease it.
2. Arrange 1 thin layer of cheese slices in the bottom of preheated waffle iron.
3. Place the beaten egg on top of the cheese.
4. Now, arrange another layer of cheese slice on top to cover evenly.
5. Cook for about 6 minutes.
6. Serve warm.

Nutrition:

- Calories: 81 Kcal
- Total Fat: 0.5 g
- Saturated Fat: 0.1 g
- Carbohydrates: 17.1 g
- Fiber: 3.4 g
- Sugars: 13 g
- Protein: 1.2 g

19. Chaffle Birthday Cake

Preparation Time: 8 minutes

Cooking Time: 16 Minutes

Servings: 2

Ingredients:

- Butter cream icing
- Birthday Cake Chaffle:
- 3 tbsp cream cheese
- 1 tbsp almond flour
- 5 tbsp coconut flour
- 1 tsp baking powder
- 6 eggs
- 2 tbsp birthday cake syrup

Directions:

1. Scoop 3 tbsp of the mixture into your waffle maker. Cook for 4 minutes and set aside.
2. Repeat the process until you have 4 cake chaffles.
3. Just like a normal cake, start assembling your cake by placing one chaffle at the bottom as the base and add a butter cream icing layer. Repeat the same process.
4. Pipe your cake edges with the icing and pile colorful shredded coconut at the center.
5. Once all the layers are completed, top with more icing and shredded coconut sprinkles.
6. Enjoy!

Nutrition:

- Calories: 131 Kcal
- Total Fat: 0.6 g
- Saturated Fat: 0.2 g
- Carbohydrates: 28.8 g
- Fiber: 6.7 g
- Sugars: 22.3 g
- Protein: 1.3 g

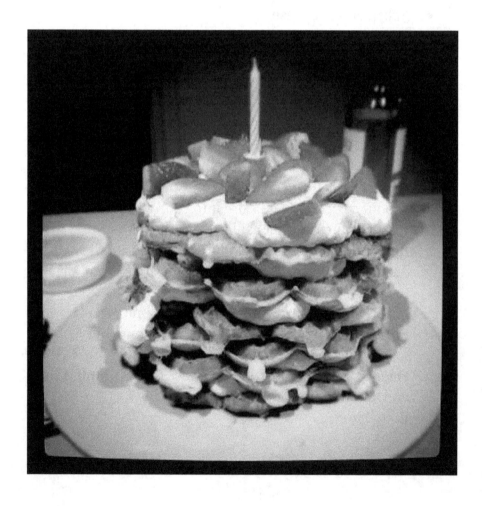

20. Chaffle-Churros

Preparation Time: 5 minutes

Cooking Time: 5 Minutes

Servings: 2

Ingredients:

- 1 egg
- 1 Tbsp almond flour
- ½ tsp vanilla extract
- 1 tsp cinnamon, divided
- ¼ tsp baking powder
- ½ cup shredded mozzarella
- 1 Tbsp swerve confectioners' sugar substitute
- 1 Tbsp swerve brown sugar substitute
- 1 Tbsp butter, melted

Directions:

1. Turn on waffle maker to heat and oil it with cooking spray.
2. Mix egg, flour, vanilla extract, ½ tsp cinnamon, baking powder, mozzarella, and sugar substitute in a bowl.
3. Place half of the mixture into waffle maker and cook for 5 minutes, or until desired doneness.
4. Remove and place the second half of the batter into the maker.
5. Cut chaffles into strips.
6. Place strips in a bowl and cover with melted butter.
7. Mix brown sugar substitute and the remaining cinnamon in a bowl.
8. Pour sugar mixture over the strips and toss to coat them well.

Nutrition:

- Protein: 61g
- Fiber:1g
- Cholesterol: 115mg
- Saturated fats: 2g
- Calories: 380

21. Strawberry Chaffle

Preparation Time: 5 minutes

Cooking Time: 8 Minutes

Servings: 2

Ingredients:

- 1 organic egg, beaten
- ¼ cup Mozzarella cheese, shredded
- 1 tablespoon cream cheese, softened
- ¼ teaspoon organic baking powder
- 1 teaspoon organic strawberry extract
- 2 fresh strawberries, hulled and sliced

Directions:

1. Preheat a mini waffle iron and then grease it.
2. In a bowl, place all ingredients except strawberry slices and beat until well combined.
3. Fold in the strawberry slices.
4. Place half of the mixture into preheated waffle iron and cook for about minutes or until golden brown.
5. Repeat with the remaining mixture.
6. Serve warm.

Nutrition:

- Protein: 56g
- Fiber: 4g
- Total carbs: 11g
- Sodium: 650mg
- Cholesterol: 145mg
- Saturated fat: 2.5g
- Total fat: 12g
- Calories: 380

22. Glazed Chaffles

Preparation Time: 5 minutes

Cooking Time: 5 Minutes

Servings: 2

Ingredients:

- ½ cup mozzarella shredded cheese
- 1/8 cup cream cheese
- 2 Tbsp unflavored whey protein isolate
- 2 Tbsp swerve confectioners' sugar substitute
- ½ tsp baking powder
- ½ tsp vanilla extract
- 1 egg
- For the glaze topping:
- 2 Tbsp heavy whipping cream
- 3-4 Tbsp swerve confectioners' sugar substitute
- ½ tsp vanilla extract

Directions:

1. Turn on waffle maker to heat and oil it with cooking spray.
2. In a microwave-safe bowl, mix mozzarella and cream cheese. Heat at 30 second intervals until melted and fully combined.
3. Add protein, 2 Tbsp sweetener, baking powder to cheese. Knead with hands until well incorporated.
4. Place dough into a mixing bowl and beat in egg and vanilla until a smooth batter form.
5. Put 1/3 of the batter into waffle maker, and cook for 3-minutes, until golden brown.
6. Repeat until all 3 chaffles are made.

7. Beat glaze ingredients in a bowl and pour over chaffles before serving.

Nutrition:

- Calories: 106
- Fat: 5.3 g
- Saturated fat: 1 g
- Carbohydrates: 12.6 g

23. Banana Nut Muffin

Preparation Time: 6 minutes

Cooking Time: 12 Minutes

Servings: 2

Ingredients:

- 1 egg
- 1 oz. cream cheese
- ¼ cup mozzarella cheese, shredded
- 1 teaspoon banana extract
- 2 tablespoons sweetener
- 1 teaspoon baking powder
- 4 tablespoons almond flour
- 2 tablespoons walnuts, chopped

Directions:

1. Combine all the ingredients in a bowl.
2. Turn on the waffle maker.
3. Add the batter to the waffle maker.
4. Seal and cook for minutes.
5. Open and transfer the waffle to a plate. Let cool for 2 minutes.
6. Do the same steps with the remaining mixture.

Nutrition:

- Calories: 100
- Fat: 6 g
- Saturated fat: 1 g

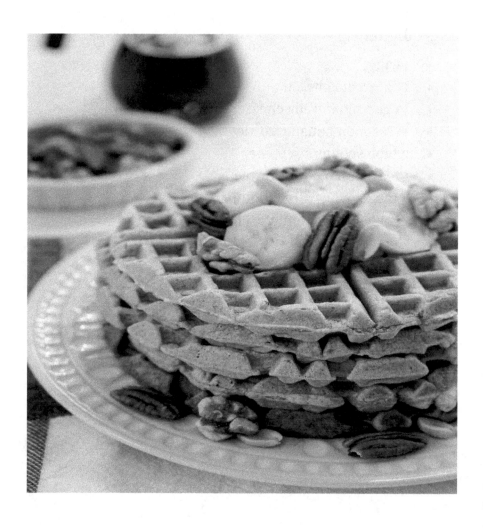

SAVORY CHAFFLE RECIPES

24. Hot Ham & Cheese Chaffles

Preparation Time: 10 minutes

Cooking Time: 5 Minutes

Servings: 2 to 3

Ingredients

- 1 large egg
- 1/2 cup of crushed swiss cheese
- 1/4 cup of deli ham, chopped
- 1/4 tsp. of garlic salt
- 1 tbsp. of mayonnaise
- 2 tsp. of Dijon mustard

Directions

1. Plug it in to preheat the waffle iron
2. Beat the egg into a bowl. And add and combine in ham, cheese and garlic salt
3. In the heated waffle iron, put half of the batter, cover it and cooking for 3-4 min or till the waffle iron finishes steaming as well as the waffle is prepared completely
4. Transfer the waffle to a tray and continue with the batter leftover
5. Mix the mustard and mayo together to use as a sauce
6. Break the waffles into half or quarters then serve with sauce

Nutrition:

- Calories: 525
- Net Carbs: 7.6 g
- Protein: 37.3 g
- Fat: 36.4 g

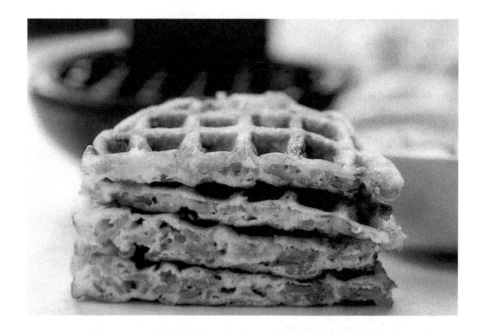

25. Big Mac Chaffle

Preparation Time: 10 minutes

Cooking Time: 10 Minutes

Servings: 2

Ingredients

- For cheeseburgers:
- 1/3 lb. of ground beef
- 1/2 tsp. of garlic salt
- 2 pieces of American cheese
- The Chaffles:
- 1 big egg
- 1/2 cup of Mozzarella finely shredded
- 1/4 tsp. of garlic salt
- For Big Mac Sauce:
- 2 tsp. of mayonnaise
- 1 tsp. of ketchup
- 1 tsp. of dill pickle relish
- splash vinegar as per your taste
- To assemble:
- 2 tbsp. of chopped lettuce
- 3 to 4 of dill pickles
- 2 tsp. of finely chopped onion

Directions

1. Making the Burgers
2. Over a mid/high heat, heat the griddle
3. Split the beef into two spheres of similar size and put each, at about 6 inches away, on the griddle
4. Let them cooking for around 1 minute

5. Using a tiny salad plate to push the beef balls tightly, to straight down to flatten. Scatter the garlic salt
6. Cooking for 2 minutes, or when cooked half completely. Carefully turn the burgers, then spray lightly with the leftover garlic salt
7. Keep cooking for 2 min or till cooked completely
8. Put one cheese slice on each patty, then pile the patties onto a plate & set aside. Wrap in foil
9. To make the chaffles:
10. Heat and spray the waffle iron with non-stick cooking oil spray
11. Mix the cheese, egg and garlic salt together until well mixed
12. In waffle iron, insert half egg mixture then cooking for 2 to 3 minutes. Place aside and replicate the step with batter left over
13. Making Big Mac Sauce:
14. Mix all items together
15. To organize burgers:
16. With stacked patties, chopped lettuce, onions, and pickle, top one chaffle
17. Scatter the Big Mac sauce on the other chaffle, then put sauce on the sandwich face down
18. Eat right away

Nutrition:

- Calories: 353
- Net Carbs: 12.9 g
- Fat: 16.3 g
- Protein: 50.3 g

26. Japanese Style Chaffle Pizza

Preparation Time: 12 minutes

Cooking Time: 6 minutes

Servings: 2

Ingredients:

- Crust
- Mozzarella cheese: 1 cup (shredded)
- Egg: 2
- Toppings
- Pizza sauce: 4 tablespoons
- Japanese sausage: 2 wholes
- Asparagus: 2 stalks
- Mozzarella cheese: 2 tablespoons (shredded)
- Kewpie mayo: 2 tablespoons
- Dried seaweed: 2 teaspoons

Directions:

1. Quickly, preheat a mini-sized waffle and grease it.
2. Using a mixing bowl, a mixture containing beaten eggs with Mozzarella cheese, mix evenly and pour into the lower side of the waffle maker.
3. With close lid, cool for 5 minutes to a crunch.
4. Preheat an oven to 500F, with the chaffle on a baking tray, pizza topping by adding the Asparagus and Japanese sausage into ¼ inch.
5. Spread the sliced asparagus, Japanese sausage and kewpie mayo on the pizza sauce on the chaffle.
6. Bake in the oven for 4 minutes at 500F until cheese melts.

7. Garnish on the top with shredded dried seaweed and enjoy.

Nutrition:

- Calories: 414
- Net Carbs: 0.3 g
- Fat: 35.2 g
- Protein: 26.7 g

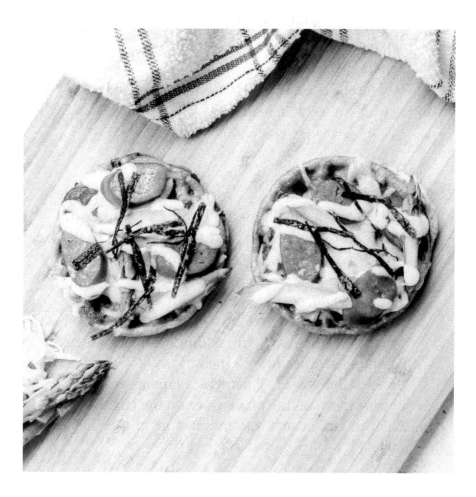

27. Keto Pepperoni Chaffle Pizza

Preparation Time: 18 minutes

Cooking Time: 12 minutes

Servings: 2

Ingredients:

- Toppings
- Tomato sauce: 2 teaspoons (sugar-free)
- Pepperoni slices: 8
- Mozzarella cheese: ½ cup shredded
- Pizza Chaffles
- Eggs: 2
- Italian season: ¼ teaspoon
- Cheddar cheese: ½ cup
- Parmesan cheese: 2 tablespoons

Directions

1. Preheat and grease a waffle maker. a combined mixture of all Pizza chaffles ingredients, evenly mixed and pour into the base of waffle maker evenly and spread.
2. With closed lids, cooking for 4 minutes till chaffles turn crispy, and then set aside.
3. Transfer the chaffle into a parchment paper-lined up.
4. Pour some tomato sauce with pepperoni sauce on each chaffle and sprinkle with shredded mozzarella.
5. Bake the chaffle in the oven for 2 minutes until the cheese turns light brown.

Nutrition:

- Calories: 246
- Total Fat: 7.4 g
- Saturated: Fat 4.6 g
- Cholesterol: 105 mg
- Total Carbs: 9.4 g
- Sugar: 6.5 g
- Fiber: 2.7 g
- Sodium: 353 mg
- Potassium: 529 mg
- Protein: 37.2 g

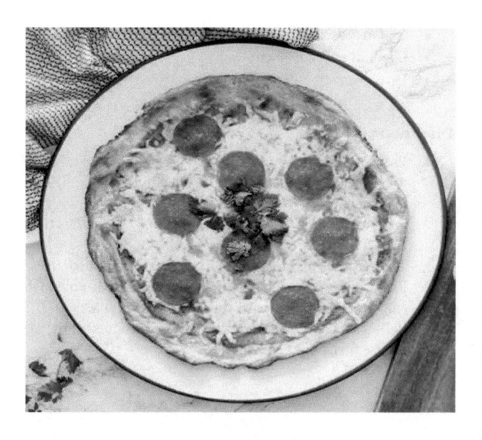

28. Keto Cauliflower Onion Pizza Chaffle

Preparation Time: 18 minutes

Cooking Time: 12 minutes

Servings: 2

Ingredients

- Toppings
- Tomato sauce: 2 teaspoons (sugar-free)
- Butter: 1 tablespoon
- Cauliflower: 4 tablespoons (diced)
- Mozzarella cheese: ½ cup shredded
- Onion: 4 tablespoons (diced)
- Salt: a pinch
- Pizza Chaffles
- Eggs: 2
- Italian season: ¼ teaspoon
- Cheddar cheese: ½ cup
- Parmesan cheese: 2 tablespoons

Directions

1. Heat some butter in a saucepan with cauliflower, heat and stir for 4 minutes.
2. Add in onions and stir for 3 minutes more, then keep aside. Preheat and grease a waffle maker.
3. Combined mixture of all Pizza chaffles ingredients, evenly mixed and pour into the base of waffle maker evenly and spread.
4. With closed lids, cooking for 7 minutes till chaffles turn crispy, and then set aside.
5. Transfer the chaffle into a parchment paper-lined up.

6. Pour some tomato sauce with onion and diced cauliflower on each chaffle and sprinkle with shredded Mozzarella cheese.
7. Bake the chaffle in the oven for 2 minutes until the cheese turns light brown.
8. Serve.

Nutrition:

- Calories: 293
- Total Fat: 16 g
- Saturated Fat: 2.3 g
- Cholesterol: 75 mg
- Total Carbs: 5.2 g
- Sugar: 2.6 g
- Fiber: 1.9 g
- Sodium: 386 mg
- Potassium: 907 mg
- Protein: 34.2 g

29.   BBQ Chicken Pizza Chaffle

Preparation Time: 18 minutes

Cooking Time: 12 minutes

Servings: 2

Ingredients

- Toppings
- Tomato sauce: 2 teaspoons (sugar-free)
- Mozzarella cheese: ½ cup shredded
- Pizza Chaffles
- Eggs: 2
- Italian season: ¼ teaspoon
- Cheddar cheese: ½ cup
- Parmesan cheese: 2 tablespoons
- BBQ Chicken
- Butter 1 tablespoon
- Chicken: ½ cup
- BBQ sauce: 1 tablespoon (sugar-free)

Directions

1. Heat some butter in a saucepan with diced chicken, heat using medium-low heat and stir for 9 minutes.
2. Add BBQ sauce, and then keep aside.
3. Preheat and grease a waffle maker. a combined mixture of all Pizza chaffles ingredients, evenly mixed and pour into the base of waffle maker evenly and spread.
4. With closed lids, cooking for 7 minutes till chaffles turns crispy, and then set aside.
5. Transfer the chaffle into a parchment paper-lined up.
6. Pour some tomato sauce with 5/6 chicken cubes on each chaffle and sprinkle with shredded Mozzarella cheese.

7. Bake the chaffle in the oven for 2 minutes until the cheese turns light brown.
8. Serve.

Nutrition:

- Calories: 457
- Total Fat: 19.1 g
- Saturated Fat: 11 g
- Cholesterol: 262 mg
- Total Carbs: 8.9 g
- Sugar: 1.2 g
- Fiber: 1.7 g
- Sodium: 557 mg
- Potassium: 748 mg
- Protein: 32.5 g

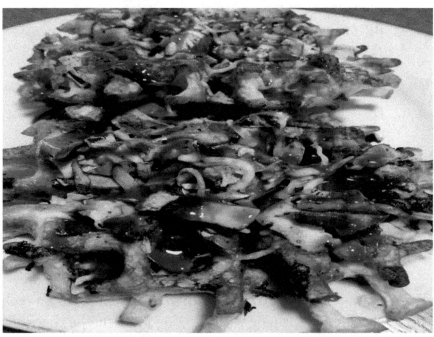

30. <u>Simple Vegetable Pizza Chaffle</u>

Preparation Time: 28 minutes

Cooking Time: 18 minutes

Servings: 2

Ingredients

- Toppings
- Tomato sauce: 2 teaspoons (sugar-free)
- Cauliflower: 4 tablespoons (diced)
- Mozzarella cheese: ½ cup shredded
- Onion: 4 tablespoons (diced)
- Olives: 4 tablespoons (diced)
- Red pepper: 4 tablespoons (diced)
- Tomatoes: 4 tablespoons (diced)
- Butter: 1 tablespoon
- Salt: a pinch
- Pizza Chaffles
- Eggs: 2
- Italian season: ¼ teaspoon
- Cheddar cheese: ½ cup
- Parmesan cheese: 2 tablespoons

Directions

1. Heat some butter in a saucepan with the vegetables (onion, tomatoes, cauliflower, red pepper) and salt for 3 minutes and keep aside.
2. Preheat and grease a waffle maker. a combined mixture of all Pizza chaffles ingredients, evenly mixed and pour into the base of waffle maker evenly and spread.
3. With closed lids, cooking for 4 minutes till chaffles turn crispy, and then set aside.

4. Transfer the chaffle into a parchment paper-lined up.
5. Pour some tomato sauce with the vegetable mixture on each chaffle and sprinkle with shredded Mozzarella cheese.
6. Bake the chaffle in the oven for 2 minutes until the cheese turns light brown.
7. The dish is ready.

Nutrition:

- Calories: 338
- Total Fat: 3.8 g
- Saturated Fat: 0.7 g
- Cholesterol: 22 mg
- Total Carbs: 8.3 g
- Fiber: 2.4 g
- Sugar: 1.2 g
- Sodium: 620 mg
- Potassium: 271 mg
- Protein: 15.4g

31. Simple Savory Chaffles

Preparation Time: 5 minutes

Cooking Time: 8 minutes

Servings: 2

Ingredients:

- 1 large organic egg, beaten
- ½ cup Cheddar cheese, shredded
- Pinch of salt and freshly ground black pepper

Directions:

1. Preheat a mini waffle iron and then grease it.
2. In a bowl, place all the ingredients and beat until well combined.
3. Place half of the mixture into preheated waffle iron and cooking for about 3-4 minutes or until golden brown.
4. Repeat with the remaining mixture.
5. Serve warm.

Nutrition:

- Calories: 604
- Total Fat: 30.6 g
- Saturated Fat: 13.1 g
- Cholesterol: 131 mg
- Total Carbs: 1.4g
- Fiber: 0.2 g
- Sugar: 20.3 g
- Sodium: 834 mg
- Potassium: 512 mg
- Protein: 54.6 g

32. Hot Pork Chaffles

Preparation Time: 10 minutes

Cooking Time: 10 minutes

Servings: 4

Ingredients:

- 1 cup pulled pork, cooked
- 2 tablespoons parmesan, grated
- 2 eggs, whisked
- 2 red chilies, minced
- 1 cup almond milk
- 1 cup almond flour
- 2 tablespoons coconut oil, melted
- 1 teaspoon baking powder

Directions:

1. In a bowl, mix the pulled pork with the eggs, parmesan and the other ingredients and whisk well.
2. Heat up the waffle maker, pour ¼ of the chaffle mix, cooking for 8 minutes and transfer to a plate.
3. Repeat with the rest of the mix and serve.

Nutrition:

- Net Carbs: 0.1g
- Calories: 110.7
- Total Fat: 8g
- Saturated Fat: 1.2g
- Protein: 9.4g
- Carbs: 0.3g
- Fiber: 0.2g
- Sugar: 0.2g

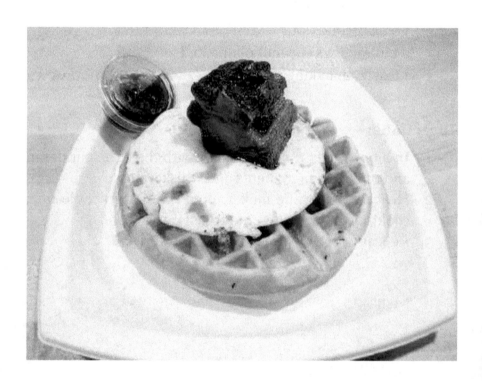

MORE KETO CHAFFLE RECIPES

33. Crispy Bacon Chaffle

Preparation Time: 5 minutes

Cooking Time: 10 minutes

Servings: 2

Ingredients:

- Cheddar cheese: 1/3 cup
- Egg: 1
- Baking powder: 1/4 teaspoon
- Flaxseed: 1 tsp. (ground)
- Parmesan cheese: 1/3 cup
- Bacon piece: 2 tbsp.

Directions:

1. Cooking the bacon pieces separately in the pan
2. Mix cheddar cheese, egg, baking powder, and flaxseed to it
3. In your mini waffle iron, shred half of the parmesan cheese
4. Grease your waffle iron lightly
5. Add the mixture from the step one to your mini waffle iron
6. Again, shred the remaining cheddar cheese on the mixtures
7. Cooking till the desired crisp is achieved
8. Make as many chaffles as your mixture and waffle maker allow

Nutrition:

- Calories: 207
- Total Fat: 4g
- Saturated Fat: 0g
- Cholesterol: 168mg
- Sodium: 536mg
- Total Carbohydrates: 5g
- Dietary Fiber: 1g
- Protein: 32g
- Sugars: 0g

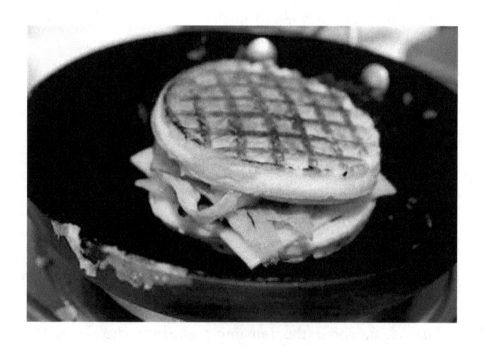

34. Almonds Crispy Chaffle

Preparation Time: 15 minutes

Cooking Time: 20 minutes

Servings: 4

Ingredients:

- Cheddar cheese: 1/3 cup
- Egg: 1
- Almond flour: 2 tbsp.
- Baking powder: 1/4 teaspoon
- Ground almonds: 2 tbsp.
- Mozzarella cheese: 1/3 cup

Directions:

1. Mix cheddar cheese, egg, almond flour, almond ground, and baking powder together in a bowl
2. Preheat your waffle iron and grease it
3. In your mini waffle iron, shred half of the Mozzarella cheese
4. Add the mixture to your mini waffle iron
5. Again, shred the remaining Mozzarella cheese on the mixture
6. Cooking till the desired crisp is achieved
7. Make as many chaffles as your mixture and waffle maker allow

Nutrition:

- Calories: 107
- Total Fat: 3g
- Saturated Fat: 0g
- Cholesterol: 8mg
- Sodium: 200mg
- Total Carbohydrates: 15g
- Dietary Fiber: 2g
- Protein: 5g
- Sugars: 0g

35. Olives Layered Chaffle

Preparation Time: 15 minutes

Cooking Time: 20 minutes

Servings: 4

Ingredients:

- For the Chaffle:
- Egg: 3
- Mozzarella cheese: 1 1/2 cup (shredded)
- Garlic powder: ½ tsp.
- Italian seasoning: 1 tsp.
- For the Vegetable:
- Mushrooms: 1 cup
- Garlic powder: ½ tsp.
- Italian seasoning: 1/2 tsp.
- Butter: 1 tbsp.
- For Layering:
- Mozzarella cheese: ½ cup (shredded)
- Olives: ½ cup
- Parsley: 1 tbsp.
- Oregano: 1 tbsp.

Directions:

1. Preheat a mini waffle maker if needed and grease it
2. In a mixing bowl, add all the ingredients of the chaffle and mix well
3. Pour the mixture to the waffle maker
4. Cooking for at least 4 minutes to get the desired crunch and make as many chaffles as your batter allows
5. In the meanwhile, melt butter and add all mushrooms ingredients and cooking

6. Remove the chaffles from the heat and spread on the baking sheet
7. Spread the cooked mushrooms on the top and sprinkle cheese and olives
8. Top again with chaffles, then mushrooms, then cheese and olives, then again chaffles and make as many layers as you want using this layering technique
9. Bake for 5 minutes in an oven at 350 degrees to melt the cheese
10. Sprinkle parsley and oregano on the top and serve hot

Nutrition:

- Calories: 395
- Fat: 2g
- Carbs: 61g
- Protein: 33g
- Fiber: 5g,
- Potassium: 796mg
- Sodium: 215 mg

36. Cin-Cheese Chaffles with the Sauce

Preparation Time: 5 minutes

Cooking Time: 15 minutes

Servings: 2

Ingredients:

- For the Chaffle:
- Egg: 1
- Mozzarella cheese: ½ cup shredded
- Cinnamon: ½ tsp.
- For the sauce:
- Mayonnaise: 1/4 cup
- Vinegar: 1 tsp.
- Sweet chili sauce: 3 tbsp.
- Hot sauce: 1 tbsp.

Directions:

1. Add egg, cinnamon, and cheese in a bowl and whisk
2. Preheat your mini waffle iron if needed and grease it
3. Cooking your mixture in the mini waffle iron for at least 4 minutes
4. Make as many chaffles as you can
5. Combine the sauce ingredient well together

Nutrition:

- Calories: 215
- Fat: 11g
- Carbs: 7g
- Protein: 24g
- Fiber: 2g
- Potassium: 520mg
- Sodium: 200mg

37. Fried Pickle Chaffle

Preparation Time: 5 minutes

Cooking Time: 10 minutes

Servings: 2

Ingredients:

- Egg: 1
- Mozzarella cheese: ½ cup (shredded)
- Pork panko: ½ cup
- Pickle slices: 6-8 thin
- Pickle juice: 1 tbsp.

Directions:

1. Mix all the ingredients well together
2. Pour a thin layer on a preheated waffle iron
3. Remove any excess juice from pickles
4. Add pickle slices and pour again more mixture over the top
5. Cooking the chaffle for around 5 minutes
6. Make as many chaffles as your mixture and waffle maker allow
7. Serve hot!

Nutrition:

- Calories: 509
- Fat: 5g
- Carbs: 69g
- Protein: 48g
- Fiber: 7g
- Potassium: 629mg
- Sodium: 400mg

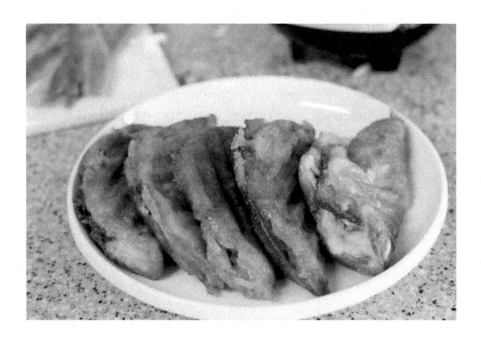

38. Plain BBQ Crispy Chaffle

Preparation Time: 5 minutes

Cooking Time: 10 minutes

Servings: 2

Ingredients:

- Cheddar cheese: 1/3 cup
- Egg: 1
- BBQ sauce: 1 tbsp.
- Baking powder: 1/4 teaspoon
- Flaxseed: 1 tsp. (ground)
- Parmesan cheese: 1/3 cup

Directions:

1. Mix cheddar cheese, egg, baking powder, BBQ sauce, and flaxseed in a bowl
2. In your mini waffle iron, shred half of the parmesan cheese
3. Grease your waffle iron lightly
4. Add the cheese mixture to the mini waffle iron
5. Again, shred the remaining parmesan cheese on the mixture
6. Cooking till the desired crisp is achieved
7. Make as many chaffles as your mixture and waffle maker allow

Nutrition:

- Calories: 434
- Fat: 16g
- Carbs: 27g
- Protein: 39g
- Fiber: 4g
- Potassium: 714mg
- Sodium: 378mg

39. Bagel Chaffles

Preparation Time: 5 minutes

Cooking Time: 10 minutes

Servings: 2

Ingredients:

- Eggs: 1
- Mozzarella cheese: ½ cup shredded
- Coconut flour: 1 tsp.
- Everything Bagel seasoning: 1 tsp.
- Cream cheese: 2 tbsp. – for serving

Directions:

1. Add all the chaffle ingredients in a bowl and whisk
2. Preheat your mini waffle iron if needed and grease it
3. Cooking your mixture in the mini waffle iron for at least 4 minutes
4. Make as many chaffles as you can and spread cream cheese on top

Nutrition:

- Calories: 311
- Fat: 13g
- Carbs: 27g
- Protein: 14g
- Fiber: 12g
- Potassium: 911mg
- Sodium: 600mg

40. Celery and Cottage Cheese Chaffles

Preparation Time: 9 minutes

Cooking Time: 15 Minutes

Servings: 4

Ingredients:

- Batter
- 4 eggs
- 2 cups grated cheddar cheese
- 1 cup fresh celery, chopped
- Salt and pepper to taste
- 2 tablespoons chopped almonds
- 2 teaspoons baking powder
- Other
- 2 tablespoons cooking spray to brush the waffle maker
- ¼ cup cottage cheese for serving

Directions:

1. Preheat the waffle maker.
2. Add the eggs, grated mozzarella cheese, chopped celery, salt and pepper, chopped almonds and baking powder to a bowl.
3. Mix with a fork.
4. Brush the heated waffle maker with cooking spray and add a few tablespoons of the batter.
5. Close the lid and cook for about 7 minutes depending on your waffle maker.
6. Serve each chaffle with cottage cheese on top.

Nutrition:

- Calories: 313
- Total Fat: 21.5g
- Saturated: Fat 9.5g
- Cholesterol: 85mg
- Sodium: 221mg
- Total Carbohydrates: 5.9g
- Dietary Fiber: 0.1g
- Sugars: 3.5g
- Protein: 34.8g
- Calcium: 16mg
- Phosphorous: 107mg
- Potassium: 281mg

CONCLUSION

Chaffles is the amazing new invention you've been waiting for. It's a revolutionary, patent-pending, and 100% vegan protein bar with a thousand uses.

What are chaffles? Chaffles is a delicious new product that can be used to replace the high fat and high sugar snacks in your diet like cheese chips or chocolate bars. It's also gluten-free, vegan, non-GMO, low in sodium and preservative free! The best part is that chaffles taste just as good as candy! You'll never want anything else again after trying this life changing snack.

The combination of protein and savory chaffle taste will keep you wanting to eat more every time. Chaffles are also a great substitute for those times that you feel like having something sweet, but want something healthy with a lot of flavor.

Chaffles come in an assortment of flavors like Pecan Pie or Cherry Pie and can be served with a drizzle of your favorite nut butter or cinnamon sugar for an awesome snack. Or you can create your own combinations by mixing them up the way that makes your mouth water.

Chaffles are great for both kids and adults. They're the perfect snack to bring on a hike for an afternoon treat or to eat on a road trip or flights. Even better, they create a new way for parents to get their kids to eat protein without them even knowing what they're eating. Now if you want your children to enjoy healthy food without complaining, chaffles will be your best friend.

No matter what you eat chaffles with, it will never disappoint! Have it with chicken noodle soup or mashed potatoes for dinner or have it with salad at lunch.

Chaffle is a perfect combination for keto dieters. Besides, keto diet is always low in carbs and high in fat so chaffle is an amazing option for it.

Chaffles are very versatile and can be used as a spread for your favorite bagel or toast, or even on top of a pizza before baking it. You can also use chaffles as an ingredient for your own meals like pancakes, pies, donuts, breads and so much more!

Chaffle comes in two different flavors: savory and sweet. The savory flavor is more of a BBQ flavor while the sweet flavor is more cookie dough style. The savory chaffles are perfect for replacing things like bread and crackers, while sweet chaffles can be used as a dessert or drink! You can also add chaffle to your favorite dessert recipes for an amazing taste.

Chaffles are the most unique tasting protein bar around that is also good for you. You won't believe how good they taste until you try them for yourself. This incredible product is sure to revolutionize your snacking experience and change the way you think about eating healthy forever.

Always remember when making your own chaffle recipes, you can choose from almost any combination of things like fruits, cereals, nuts and seeds. You can even use different types of chocolate in some recipes. Anything goes with chaffle!

What's even more exciting is that chaffles come in many sizes to fit anyone's taste and diet.

It's time to ditch your unhealthy snacks for life changing chaffles!

CPSIA information can be obtained
at www.ICGtesting.com
Printed in the USA
BVHW010031270621
610445BV00014B/106